Elaine Romero Silva

Comparison between normative and self-perceived needs

Elaine Romero Silva

Comparison between normative and self-perceived needs

ScienciaScripts

Imprint

Any brand names and product names mentioned in this book are subject to trademark, brand or patent protection and are trademarks or registered trademarks of their respective holders. The use of brand names, product names, common names, trade names, product descriptions etc. even without a particular marking in this work is in no way to be construed to mean that such names may be regarded as unrestricted in respect of trademark and brand protection legislation and could thus be used by anyone.

Cover image: www.ingimage.com

This book is a translation from the original published under ISBN 978-613-9-62814-8.

Publisher:
Sciencia Scripts
is a trademark of
Dodo Books Indian Ocean Ltd. and OmniScriptum S.R.L publishing group

120 High Road, East Finchley, London, N2 9ED, United Kingdom
Str. Armeneasca 28/1, office 1, Chisinau MD-2012, Republic of Moldova, Europe
Printed at: see last page
ISBN: 978-620-7-75139-6

SUMMARY

I dedicate this work to my parents, Antônia and Evandro, to my loves Nicolas and Pietro and to my boyfriend, Fàbio, for their continuous demonstrations of unconditional love, without whose support the journey would be much more difficult. Thank you for agreeing to deprive yourselves of my company, giving me the opportunity to achieve even more.

THANKS

To Prof.ª Dr.ª **Sandra Mara Maciel** for her dedicated guidance and patience with my imperfections;

To my co-supervisor and friend **Luiz Sérgio Carreiro**, who was always willing to collaborate;

To the examining board for the exchange of ideas, suggestions and constructive discussions during the qualification and defense of this dissertation;

To the professors and colleagues in the master's program for the knowledge acquired and for their friendship;

To all those who took part in the data collection for their availability, joy and friendship, my special thanks to **Carlos Tambelini, Denise Ramos, Heliton Lima, Nicole Brunozi, Silvia Chadi and Anderson Aleixo;**

To the **Regional Education Center**, and to each school principal, for readily allowing access to the state schools;

To my colleagues **Bruno Rosa, Georges Garcia, Ricardo Zampieri and Wagner Ursi**, who, each in their own way, have shown their true friendship since our undergraduate days;

To my secretary **Michelly Souza**, for her support and words of encouragement whenever I needed them;

And to all the colleagues, friends, family and patients who shared this period of my life, for their support and patience.

For having contributed to the completion of this dissertation.

Thank you so much!

THANKS

To the **Universidade Norte do Paranà**, UNOPAR, represented by the Chancellor, **Mr. Marco Antônio Laffranchi** and the Rector, **Prof.ª . Elisabeth Bueno Laffranchi**;

To the **Dean of Research and Postgraduate Studies**, represented by **Prof. Dr. Hélio Hiroshi Suguimoto;**

To the **Center for Biological Health Sciences**, represented by **Prof. Ruy Moreira da Costa Filho**;

To the **Coordination of the Dentistry Course**, represented by **Prof. Dr. Luiz Reynaldo de Figueiredo Walter**;

To **all the staff at UNOPAR;**

For having contributed to the completion of this dissertation.

Thank you so much!

ROMERO, Elaine. **Comparison between the normative needs for orthodontic treatment and those self-perceived by adolescents in Londrina - Pr.**2008.67f. Dissertation (Master's Degree in Dentistry) Universidade Norte do Paranà, Londrina.

SUMMARY

Aesthetics play an important role in individuals' social interaction. In some situations, the presence of aligned teeth seems to have a strong influence on the perception of beauty, identification with professional success and intelligence, and is even associated with more socially advantaged individuals. Orthodontic treatments are carried out in the hope of improving the appearance and masticatory function of individuals and are generally indicated and carried out using clinical or epidemiological criteria (normative needs), i.e. based on professional decisions. However, these criteria can overestimate occlusal problems. The aim of this study was to compare the technically defined orthodontic needs (normative criteria) and the self-perceived orthodontic needs (subjective criteria) of 428 adolescents aged between 15 and 19, of both genders, from the Londrina-PR public school system. Clinical examinations were conducted to verify the presence of malocclusions (normative need for orthodontic treatment), using the diagnostic criteria established by the *Dental Aesthetic Index* (DAI), according to the World Health Organization. Socio-demographic and behavioral characteristics were obtained through personal interviews with the students. A structured interview questionnaire was used to assess the adolescents' and their parents' perception of the need for orthodontic treatment. The adolescents assessed their need for treatment using a 10 cm Visual Analogue Scale (VAS) and the examiner carried out the same process. The DAI indicators associated with the need for treatment were overjet, crowding and missing teeth. Adolescents who were dissatisfied with their smile and the appearance of their teeth represented the largest proportion of the population in need of orthodontic treatment, as evidenced by the statistical association. There was a significant association between normative and self-perceived treatment needs.

Keywords: Malocclusion - perception - normative need - orthodontic treatment

1. INTRODUCTION

In the last 40 years, there have been notable changes in the epidemiological patterns of diseases and conditions affecting oral health, with different morbidities and conditions gaining importance for public health (PERES and TOMITA, 2006). In a scale of priorities for oral problems proposed by the World Health Organization (1989), dental caries ranks first, followed by periodontal diseases and malocclusions. However, depending on the region in which the analysis is carried out and the characteristics of the population under study, tooth decay may not represent the main oral health problem and any of the other problems may become a higher priority and more relevant from the point of view of social and health significance (MOURA and CAVALCANTI, 2007).

Malocclusion is a variation of normal growth and development that affects facial muscles and bones during childhood and adolescence. Misaligned teeth can cause psychosocial problems related to dentofacial aesthetics; disturbances in oral function, such as chewing, swallowing and speech; and increased susceptibility to trauma and periodontal disease. It is common knowledge, confirmed by various epidemiological studies, that the prevalence and severity of occlusal disorders have increased over the last two hundred years, especially with regard to dental crowding (FRAZÂO and NARVAI,2006).

Occlusion assessment indices are generally not designed to quantify the need for treatment, and are usually used as the first tool to assess this need (COOPER et al. 2000).

Using Angle's classification of malocclusion, Silva Filho et al, in 1989, assessed the occlusal conditions of 2416 schoolchildren in the city of Bauru, aged between 7 and 11, from public and private schools. The results showed that only 11.4% of the population had normal occlusion. Of the malocclusions, class I prevailed (55%), followed by class II (42%) and finally class III (3%). The morphological deviations posterior crossbite (18.2%) and deep overbite (19.8%) were assessed by the authors.

Galvao, Pereira and Bello (1994) reviewed epidemiological studies of malocclusions in Latin America and found high prevalence rates, with percentages rarely below 50%.

In the latest nationwide epidemiological study on the oral health conditions of the Brazilian population (BRASIL, 2004), occlusal problems were assessed for the first time. The results showed that more than half (53.23%) of adolescents aged between 15 and 19 had a malocclusion and revealed that among these, the prevalence of very severe or disabling occlusal conditions reached 18.75%.

Over the last few decades, there has been a growing demand for orthodontic treatment, which can be attributed to a number of reasons, including a general improvement in oral health with a decline in dental caries, greater awareness and expectations regarding oral health and a greater availability of dental treatment. As a result of this demand, waiting lists for orthodontic treatment have grown (OLIVEIRA, 2004).

In childhood and adolescence, malocclusion represents problems of growth and development that affect the muscles and jawbones and can produce aesthetic changes in the teeth or face, as well as functional changes involving chewing, speech and occlusion of the teeth (SIMOES, 1978).

The main benefits of orthodontic treatment are related to an improvement in both oral function and appearance, which would lead to psychological improvement and social well-being (SANDY and ROBERTS-HARRY, 2003). Orthodontic diagnosis places little emphasis on patients' perceptions of this need and the impact that orthodontic treatment has on their quality of life (OLIVEIRA and SHEIHAM, 2003).

Children's and adolescents' feelings about their appearance or dental function should be the central focus for assessing the need for and carrying out orthodontic treatment. However, traditional methods of assessing orthodontic needs or evaluating treatments carried out are mainly based on normative needs (NN) estimated by professionals, using cephalometric or occlusal measurements to define the need for treatment or its success (BELL et al. 1985; KEROSUO, 1995; PHILIPS et al. 1995; HANCOCK and BLINKHORN, 1996; KOOCHEK et al. 2001; JOHANSSON AND FOLLIN, 2005; GHERUNPONG et al. 2006).

It is essential that orthodontists understand the importance of communicating and counseling about the need for treatment, given the different perceptions of individuals on this subject. The desire for orthodontic treatment in children is directly influenced by parental attitudes and values. Likewise, parents' decisions are partly the result of the guidance given by the orthodontist (ESPELAND et al, 1992).

As there are degrees of occlusal problems defined by the professional that are acceptable to the patient, this should be taken into account when indicating orthodontic treatment, especially in public services (DIAS et al, 2008).

Due to an arbitrary and subjective process observed in the selection of patients for orthodontic treatment, some individuals receive treatment despite the indication of lesser need, while others, with greater need, fail to receive it. One suggestion for screening these patients would be to use an occlusal index (STENVICK et al., 1997; DIAS and GLEISER,

2008).

It is clear that a method for assessing the need for orthodontic treatment requires the integration of normative clinical measures with a patient-based indicator, considering both impacts related to oral function and appearance, as well as measures of oral health behavior. In this way, orthodontic need can be more appropriately used in the planning of dental services (MANDALL et al. 1999; GHERUNPONG et al. 2006), since the need for orthodontic treatment is difficult for professionals to define precisely because deviations from "normal" occlusion are not always clear and easy to identify, i.e. it is not easy to delineate "acceptable occlusions" from "unacceptable occlusions" (MARQUES et al, 2005).

In view of the fact that traditional malocclusion assessment practices have limitations and considering the importance of individuals' self-perception and opinions for orthodontic treatment recommendations, this study was carried out. To this end, the technically defined orthodontic needs (normative criteria) were compared with the self-perceived needs (subjective criteria) of adolescents aged between 15 and 19 from public schools in Londrina-Pr.

2. LITERATURE REVIEW

The scientific literature on malocclusion is varied, ranging from clinical, physiological and socio-cultural aspects.

The classification of malocclusion is particularly important in diagnostic procedures and orthodontic treatment planning. At the end of the 19th century, Edward Hartley Angle developed a method of classifying malocclusion based on the anteroposterior relationship of the upper and lower first permanent molars. If the mid-vestibular cusp of the upper first permanent molar rested in the buccal groove of the lower first molar and if the teeth were aligned in the arches, this would be considered an ideal occlusion; if there were problems in the anterior region (overbite, anterior open bite, crowding, etc.), the malocclusion would be called class I. A class II malocclusion would present a distal deviation in this occlusion relationship, while a distal occlusion of the cusp in relation to the sulcus would be classified as class III (SALZMANN, 1968; MOYERS, 1991; PROFFIT and FIELDS, 1995).

According to Pinto et al (2008), the Angle classification has undergone changes over the years in order to minimize its shortcomings, including the failure to consider transverse problems in the assessment, as well as compromised facial aesthetics. The validity and reliability of the Angle classification for epidemiological studies has been questioned, as it is a qualitative rather than quantitative index of malocclusion.

Malocclusion can be based on cultural values (body image and aesthetics), anatomical deviations from morphological norms, well defined by the clinician, and functional considerations that impair mastication.

Grainger defined the problem of malocclusion according to one of the following components: 1) unacceptable aesthetics, 2) a significant reduction in the function of the masticatory system, 3) a traumatic condition that predisposes to tissue destruction in the form of periodontal disease or caries, 4) speech problems, 5) lack of stability in the occlusion and 6) congenital anomalies or trauma. In an epidemiological investigation, malocclusion is the only one that is not necessarily understood as an abnormality and does not always incapacitate or invalidate individuals. The boundary between acceptable and unacceptable malocclusions is influenced by psychological and social factors and, by considering people's perceptions, the aim is to overcome the limitations of normative standards and the exclusive judgment of professionals. Many orthodontic therapies are carried out for aesthetic reasons (PINTO et al. 2008).

Although epidemiological studies on the occurrence of malocclusion have been reported in various countries, it is difficult to compare them, mainly due to the lack of standardization of the indices and criteria used. At the moment, even the World Health Organization (WHO) database has limited data on this oral health problem (OLIVEIRA, 2004).

Since 1962, the WHO has advocated epidemiological surveys of occlusal conditions using simple and easy-to-use indices. Occlusal indices were developed in response to the growing demand for orthodontic treatment, with the aim of prioritizing patients according to the severity of their malocclusion and the need for treatment. According to Baume (1974), these instruments were developed to measure the prevalence of orthodontic problems in the population and to evaluate the treatments carried out, each of them separately or as a whole constituting complex observation systems.

Using Angle's classification of malocclusion, Silva Filho et al, in 1989, assessed the occlusal conditions of 2416 schoolchildren in the city of Bauru, of both genders, aged between 7 and 11, from public and private schools. The results showed that only 11.4% of the population had normal occlusion. Of the malocclusions, class I prevailed (55%), followed by class II (42%) and finally class III (3%).

Malocclusion requires a uniform assessment method that prioritizes the individuals most in need of orthodontic treatment. As the demand for this type of treatment in public services in Brazil exceeds the supply, there is a need to implement an appropriate means of selecting patients, thus facilitating referral and screening for orthodontic treatment (DIAS, 2008).

Although there is still no universally accepted index for measuring malocclusion, the World Health Organization (WHO, 1989) has recognized and indicated the *Dental Aesthetic Index* (DAI) in surveys to assess orthodontic treatment needs, as an examination tool to determine the priority for orthodontic care in public health programs.

Considering that dental appearance is the factor that motivates people to seek treatment, the DAI was proposed by Cons et al (1986). From 500,000 high school students in New York State, aged between 15 and 18, 1337 study models, representative of this population, were obtained. From these, 200 occlusal configurations were evaluated using photographs, taking into account their social acceptability. Available for each photograph were 49 anatomical measurements of occlusal features considered important in the development of the orthodontic index, which allowed aesthetic and clinical components to be linked mathematically to produce a single score combining the physical and aesthetic aspects of occlusion (JAHN, 2005).

The components of the Dental Aesthetics Index are divided into three groups: dentition, space and occlusion (CONS, 1983). Occlusion problems such as posterior crossbites, posterior open bites, deep bites, midline deviations, dental impactions and missing molars are not verified in the DAI (DANYLUK et al.1999).

Another index that is gaining increasing acceptance is the Orthodontic Treatment Needs Index (IOTN) (BROOK and SHAW, 1989). In this index, the various malocclusion problems are placed on a scale combined with another scale relating to perceptions of aesthetic inadequacies (PINTO, 2000). BROOK and SHAW (1989) assessed the need for orthodontic treatment using the IOTN. However, there is strong evidence to suggest the need for an additional social point of view (SHEIHAM et al. 1987). In general, such information provides advantages in understanding behavior related to oral health and extending oral assessment beyond the limits of epidemiological indices (SLADE and SPENCER, 1994).

For more than three decades, the importance of the aesthetic implications of malocclusion has been recognized as a significant factor in assessing the need for orthodontic treatment (HUNT et al. 2002). Smiling is of great importance, both for the individual's interaction with others and for their self-esteem (REIS et al. 1990; PATEL et al. 2007). Similarly, children who were worried about their teeth and children with missing, stained or decayed teeth were less confident about their smile (LOW et al. 1999).

Individual motivation to seek orthodontic treatment seems to be strongly associated with perceptions of how much their dentofacial appearance deviates from socio-cultural norms. From this perspective, a personal response to dentofacial attractiveness can be viewed as a type of psychosocial response to occlusal status. As such, these responses have a cultural emphasis (TEDESCO et al. 1983). In children, the desire for treatment is influenced by the attitudes and values of their parents. It is apparently recognized by both parents and children that social adaptation and chances of success increase according to facial beauty (ESPELAND et al. 1992).

It is important to note that women, older people and those from a higher social class are considered to be more critical of their dental aesthetics (DIAS et al. 2008).

Orthodontic treatments are carried out in the hope of improving the appearance and masticatory function of individuals and are generally indicated and carried out based on clinical or epidemiological criteria (normative needs), i.e. professional decisions. It is difficult to determine how important malocclusions are as a facial problem and what impact this problem has on the quality of life of affected individuals (PERES et al. 2002).

Measures of orthodontic needs place relatively little emphasis on patients' perceptions of these needs and the difference orthodontic care can make to their daily activities (OLIVEIRA and SHEIHAM, 2003).

From the patient's point of view, the main factors influencing the decision to undergo orthodontic treatment are: dissatisfaction with dentofacial appearance, recommendation by the dentist, concern on the part of parents and the influence of schoolmates who wear braces (SHAW et al. 1991). The presence of aligned teeth has a strong influence on the perception of beauty, identification with professional success and intelligence and association with more socially advantaged individuals (PERES et al. 2002).

Shaw et al. (1991) observed that children with less perceived oral care tended to be dissatisfied with their dental appearance and to perceive a greater need for orthodontic treatment. They emphasized that the decision to treat orthodontically is particularly challenging when malocclusion represents a limiting need, consisting mainly of aesthetic improvement. Consent to treatment implies a process in which the potential patient obtains sufficient information about treatment needs and alternatives to enable them to make decisions about treatment independently (NASH, 1988).

Espeland et al. (1992) assessed the perception of 93 children and their parents, as well as two orthodontists, regarding the need for orthodontic treatment. By analyzing photographs of various malocclusions, they found no significant differences between the genders or between parents and their children in relation to this concern. Severe overjet and spacing were the problems most recognized by both parents and children. There was no agreement in the recording of misalignments between parents and professionals, especially when it came to mild or moderate irregularities. They concluded that decisions about therapeutic intervention should consider the social and individual aspects of dentofacial appearance.

Peres et al. (2002) observed that the presence of incisal crowding and marked overjet were risk factors for dissatisfaction with the appearance of students aged 14 to 18 at a high school in Florianópolis. The authors sought to identify normative orthodontic treatment needs, assess their impact on satisfaction with appearance and compare them with self-perceived needs in a group of 315 adolescents. The DAI was used to diagnose the main malocclusions, and a questionnaire was used to find out the students' satisfaction with their appearance and their perception of the need for orthodontic treatment. There was a higher prevalence among males (75.6%) compared to females (68%), but this difference was not statistically significant (p=0.15).

Of all the students with normative needs, just over half (61.1%) perceived the need for orthodontic treatment. This perception was higher among adolescents with antero-lower jaw crowding ("*Odds Rate*"= 3.3), overjet (OR=1.7) and anterior diastema (OR=3.1), regardless of the presence of other malocclusions. In view of their results, the authors pointed out that there are technically defined degrees of occlusal problems that are acceptable to the population and that these can influence treatment decisions, directly interfering in the demand for this type of care.

Perin (2002), evaluating 734 twelve-year-old public schoolchildren of both genders, found 66.7% with malocclusion using Angle's classification. On the other hand, using the Dental Aesthetics Index, he found 65.2% of adolescents with no abnormality or mild malocclusion. Definite malocclusion was found in 12.8%, while severe malocclusion was observed in 10.9% and very severe or disabling malocclusion in 11.0%. Most of the children (70.5%) had normal molar relationships. The Dental Aesthetics Index was not sensitive to some occlusion problems when compared to the Angle classification.

Cunha et al. in 2003 evaluated 120 patients treated at the FOUERJ orthodontic specialization course with regard to their malocclusion, aesthetic damage and degree of need for orthodontic treatment, using the DAI and IOTN indices. They found that over 70% of the cases treated had a severe need for orthodontic treatment, according to both indices, and the most frequent occlusal characteristics were: overjet of more than 3.5mm, crowding and missing teeth.

Grzywacz (2003) examined 84 12-year-old children in order to estimate whether the dental concept expressed by the aesthetic component (AC) scale of the IOTN chosen by the schoolchildren was reliable and predictive of their potential to cooperate once they had undergone orthodontic treatment. To this end, the children completed a questionnaire and evaluated their own dentition using a color illustration of the AC during a clinical examination at school. When shown the scale with 10 photographs containing various degrees of dental attractiveness, the main question was: "Where would you place your teeth on this scale?". Although 61.9% of the children evaluated reported being satisfied with their dental aesthetics, 65.4% expressed a desire to modify some aspects of their dentition, such as alignment (55.4%) and tooth color (43%). The author emphasized the difficulty individuals have in indicating their own dentition on the AC scale, especially in the case of children. She concluded that the criterion of using this scale to assess the need for orthodontic treatment moderately reflected the self-perception in relation to dental aesthetics of the group studied.

In a study involving 1,675 adolescents, Oliveira and Sheiham (2003) looked at whether the fact of having received orthodontic treatment would affect the levels of impact on oral health-related quality of life, as well as verifying the relationship between clinical measures of the need for normative orthodontic treatment (IOTN) and two measures of oral health-related quality of life (OIDP - Index of Oral Impacts on Daily Activities and OHIP - Oral Health Impact Profile). The sample was aged between 15 and 16 and was divided into three groups according to their history of orthodontic treatment: treated, under treatment and untreated. They found that those who had received orthodontic treatment reported less impact on their daily activities than those who had not. The authors recommended that conventional methods of assessing the need for orthodontic treatment should be complemented by measures of oral health-related quality of life that would enable a psychosocial understanding of the need for orthodontic treatment.

Baca-Garcia et al, in 2004, with the aim of evaluating the prevalence of malocclusion and the need for treatment in 744 schoolchildren aged between 14 and 20, from rural and urban areas in Granada, Spain, found 41.4% of malocclusion. There was no significant difference in DAI scores between the rural and urban populations, but a statistical difference was found between social classes, with the least advantaged having the worst scores.

Hamdan, in 2004, studying a sample of 103 patients with an average age of 15, compared the responses of these patients with those given by their parents, with the aim of observing the perceived needs of parents, patients and clinicians, using the IOTN index. The majority of patients (93%) emphasized aesthetics as the main factor in their decision to seek orthodontic treatment. Parents' desire for treatment for their children was greater than that of adolescents. He observed that the desire for orthodontic treatment is multifactorial and influenced by elements other than normative ones and the perception of aesthetics. For him, the factors that contribute to these differences are: social class, economic considerations, individual perceptions of psychosocial benefits and behavior in relation to the use of orthodontic appliances.

In 2004, Reyes et al. evaluated 176 adolescents under the age of 19 in Santa Clara, Cuba, with the aim of showing the clinical state of dental occlusion using the DAI. Clinical dental examinations were carried out by a specialist and individual interviews. There was agreement in most cases between the normative and subjective criteria, especially in very severe malocclusions. The authors reported a 96% sensitivity of the index with regard to the need for priority treatment, when compared to the orthodontist's analysis, with 38.1%

of malocclusion present, 13.6% of which was severe or disabling. However, they highlight its low sensitivity and specificity in cases where elective treatment is needed (definite malocclusion). When analyzing the dependent variable satisfaction with dental appearance, they observed a significant causal relationship with dental crowding, increasing the risk of dissatisfaction in adolescents fourfold (OR= 4.21).

Analyzing the distribution of malocclusion in the population of the state of São Paulo, using data from the epidemiological survey on the oral conditions of the Brazilian population (BRASIL, 2004), Jahn (2005) observed that the prevalence of definite malocclusion was 13%, severe malocclusion 6% and disabling malocclusion 6% for the group studied with the DAI. There was a significantly higher percentage of severe or disabling malocclusion in the rural population compared to the urban population and in black and brown schoolchildren compared to white schoolchildren. There was no significant difference between the rates of very severe or disabling malocclusion among male and female schoolchildren, and between public and private schoolchildren.

Marques et al. (2005) studied 333 schoolchildren aged 10 to 14 in Belo Horizonte, with the aim of verifying the association between normative orthodontic treatment needs and psychosocial aspects. To this end, they used the clinical criteria recommended by the DAI and a questionnaire addressed to parents and adolescents. They observed that the desire for orthodontic treatment reported by the adolescents and the parents' perception of their child's oral aesthetics showed a significant correlation with the normative need for this type of treatment. The prevalence of malocclusion was 62%, 62.6% in 10 to 12-year-olds and 61.3% in 13 to 14-year-olds. Orthodontic treatment was considered necessary in 174 schoolchildren (52.3%). In 86 (25.8%), it was considered elective and for the same frequency of adolescents, this treatment was considered highly desirable (13.2%) and essential (13.2%). The majority of schoolchildren reported that they wished to be treated orthodontically (87.7%), while 82.9% of parents believed that their children needed orthodontic treatment. Socio-demographic indicators such as mother's schooling, economic level, age and gender of the children were not statistically associated with the normative need for orthodontic treatment. The most frequent types of malocclusion were crowding greater than or equal to 2mm in one or two segments (37.8%) and overjet greater than or equal to 4mm (37.5%). The authors drew attention to the importance of incorporating psychosocial factors into orthodontic treatment decisions.

Onyeaso and Sanu in 2005, when investigating the possible relationship between concern about malocclusion among Nigerian adolescents, their satisfaction with their dental appearance and the severity of their occlusal irregularities, as measured by the DAI, found no statistically significant difference between the genders. On the other hand, they observed a significant negative correlation between the different levels of malocclusion severity (normative need for treatment) and satisfaction with appearance.

Frazao and Narvai, in 2006, evaluated 13801 children and adolescents aged between 12 and 18 in the state of Sao Paulo, with the aim of verifying the prevalence and severity of malocclusion using the DAI, and found a prevalence of 16.5% of severe or very severe malocclusion. Moderate malocclusion was more frequent among older individuals. The most frequent problems were the presence of spacing in one of the arches in the anterior region, interincisor diastemas and maxillary overjet. They concluded that 1 in 6 of them needed orthodontic treatment, in a proportion of 73% of public school children compared to private school children, and only 11% were white.

With the aim of evaluating the aesthetic impact of malocclusion on the daily lives of Brazilian schoolchildren and testing the association between the aesthetic impact of malocclusion and biopsychosocial variables, Marques et al (2006) observed 333 schoolchildren aged between 10 and 14 with no history of orthodontic treatment. The measure used was the aesthetic impact of malocclusion on the schoolchildren's daily activities (OIDP). The criterion used to determine the normative need for treatment was the DAI. Self-perception was assessed using the Oral Aesthetics Subjective Impact Scale (OASIS). The results showed that 27% of the schoolchildren reported an aesthetic impact on their daily activities due to malocclusion, and there was a statistical association between these two variables. Risk factors for esthetic impact were: female gender, anterior-superior crowding of 2mm or more, normative need for treatment considered elective and highly desirable, negative self-perception of oral esthetics, low self-esteem and intermediate economic level.

Santos, in 2006, assessed the reliability of the DAI in a sample of 120 adult patients aged between 19 and 78 using study models, photographs and a questionnaire. Thirty-three orthodontists took part in the study and determined whether or not orthodontic treatment was necessary, classifying it into four categories: none, little, medium or great need. According to the severity of malocclusion, the prevalence was distributed as follows: 16.7% equal to definite malocclusion; 26.7%, severe and 48.3%, very severe. The study found that the DAI index was accurate in assessing the severity of malocclusion and the need for orthodontic treatment, and that patients had a low rate of self-perception of this need. Orthodontic treatment was considered necessary in 75% of patients. The subjective assessment of the need for treatment by specialists proved to be of low accuracy or reliability. As for the types of malocclusion, anterior-inferior misalignment and dental crowding were the most prevalent, with 80% and 75.9%, respectively.

Moura and Cavalcanti in 2007, when assessing 400 12-year-old schoolchildren in Campina Grande-PA, with the aim of verifying adolescents' perceptions of satisfaction when smiling and difficulty chewing food, in an attempt to correlate them with the severity of malocclusion, observed a discrepancy between the schoolchildren's perceptions and the normative values for malocclusion. According to the normative criteria (DAI), orthodontic treatment was considered necessary in 78.4% of the schoolchildren. Treatment of malocclusion was considered elective in 23.8% of schoolchildren, while treatment was considered highly desirable and essential in 18.2% and 36.4% of schoolchildren respectively.

Peres et al. in 2008, evaluating 900 15-year-old adolescents with the aim of assessing whether malocclusion had an impact on their satisfaction with their appearance, found that severe/moderate malocclusion had an impact on adolescent girls' satisfaction with their appearance, even when other physical characteristics were taken into account. This pattern was not observed in boys. The boys were more concerned about their physical constitution, unlike the girls, who were concerned about a number of other aspects, such as the presence of malocclusion. One interpretation of this difference between the sexes is that female attractiveness standards are much higher than male ones in a broad cultural context. The prevalence of moderate or severe malocclusion was 58.8% and normal or mild malocclusion, 40.5%.

Pinheiro et al. 2008, in their studies carried out in Natal and Joâo Pessoa, compared the perception of the need for treatment between 57 patients, with an average age of 14 years, and 31 orthodontists using only illustrations of some characteristics of malocclusions, and highlighted that diastema was equally perceived by patients and professionals in the two cities studied, with orthodontic correction being indicated in both groups. In Natal, antero-lower crowding was diagnosed more by professionals than by patients, but the need for treatment was pointed out by both groups. In Joâo Pessoa, on the other hand, patients and professionals equally recognized antero-inferior crowding, although the latter showed greater interest in orthodontic correction. As expected, midline deviation was more noticeable to professionals in both cities. Of those professionals and patients who recognized this alteration, approximately half indicated orthodontic treatment, which highlights the importance of discussing the intention and feasibility of correcting it with patients. The authors considered overbite to be the most worrying malocclusion for patients.

3. OBJECTIVES

3.1 General Objective:

- To compare the technically defined orthodontic needs (normative criteria) with the self-perceived needs (subjective criteria) of adolescents aged 15 to 19 from public schools in Londrina-PR and their guardians.

3.2 Specific objectives:

•	To determine the prevalence of malocclusion according to Angle's classification and the normative orthodontic treatment needs (DAI) of adolescents aged 15 to 19 from public schools in Londrina, PR,

•	To assess the perception of adolescents and their guardians regarding their need for orthodontic treatment.

•	Checking for an association between socio-demographic factors and normative and perceived orthodontic treatment needs

4. MATERIAL AND METHOD

3.3 Study design

This is a cross-sectional observational study conducted to compare the perceptions or needs expressed by adolescents in relation to orthodontic treatment with the normative needs.

3.4 Geographical location of the study

This study was conducted in Londrina - Paranà, which has 495,696 inhabitants (IBGE, 2006), from different social strata.

3.5 Study population

The universe of this study was made up of students aged between 15 and 19, of both genders, from the Londrina-PR state public school system.

According to the school census published by the Regional Education Center, at the beginning of 2008, 23,213 students were enrolled in secondary school, 78.71% of them in the Londrina public school system.

The sample size was calculated considering a 95% confidence interval and a tolerable margin of error of 5%, using the formula proposed by Barbetta (2007).

TABLE 1 - Formula for calculating the minimum sample size.

	Being:
$$n_0 = \frac{1}{(E_0)^2}$$ $$n = \frac{N \times n_0}{N + n_0}$$	n_0 - dimensioned sample number And_0 - margin of error 5% N - Population size n - Sample size

From the total of 18,273, a minimum sample size of 391 schoolchildren was defined. To compensate for any losses, 20% (N=469) was added to the sample.

In order to obtain the study population, a random sampling technique was used, which obeyed the following criteria: a) Dividing the city into 5 geographical regions (North, South, East, West and Central); b) Within each region, after classifying the schools by student size, two schools were drawn, one small and one large; c) drawing classes from 1[a]. to 3. [a]to the 3rd grade of secondary education; d) drawing of lots for students aged 15 to 19, in numbers proportional to the size of the school.

3.6 Preliminary procedures

As determined by the National Health Council, this study was submitted to the Standing Committee on Ethics and Research Involving Human Beings of the Universidade Norte do Paranà - UNOPAR, under protocol number 0012/08 (Annex A).

After obtaining official authorization from the Londrina Regional Education Office for the research to be carried out (Appendix B), official authorization was sought from the management of the schools selected (Appendix C). And through

A list of enrolled students was provided, a draw was made and the Terms of Free and Informed Consent were sent to their guardians (Appendix D).

3.7 Occlusal condition assessment

The Dental Aesthetic Index (DAI) was used to assess dentofacial abnormalities in schoolchildren. The components of the Dental Aesthetic Index are divided into three groups: **dentition**, determined by the number of missing teeth in the anterior region; **space**, which is based on the presence or absence of crowding and spacing, the existence or not of diastema between upper central incisors and upper and lower misalignment; and finally, the **occlusion** group with the components - upper and lower dental projection; anterior open bite and anteroposterior molar relationship (CONS, 1983).The DAI is a logistic regression equation that mathematically relates the public's perception of dental aesthetics with objective physical measurements of occlusal characteristics associated with malocclusion (Chart 2). To do this, the 10 components are measured in each individual to obtain each numerical value, each numerical value is multiplied by its corresponding standard DAI regression coefficient and the values obtained are added to a constant 13. The result corresponds to the DAI value.

Table 2. Occlusal components considered in the standard Dental Aesthetic Index (DAI) and respective regression coefficients.

COMPONENTS OF DAI	WEIGHTS
DENTIATION	6
CROWDING IN THE INCISAL SEGMENT	1
SPACING IN THE INCISAL SEGMENT	1
INCISAL DIASTEMA	3
ANTERIOR MAXILLARY MISALIGNMENT	1
ANTERIOR MANDIBULAR MISALIGNMENT	1
SPARE	4
ANTERIOR CROSSBITE	4
ANTERIOR OPEN BITE	4

ANTEROPOSTERIOR MOLAR RATIO	3
CONSTANT	13
	SCORE
TOTAL	**DAI**

Both the severity of malocclusion and the need for treatment are classified based on the scores obtained, as shown in Table 3.

Chart 3 - Distribution of standard DAI values according to severity of malocclusion and indication for treatment.

Severity of malocclusion	Indication of treatment	DAI score
No abnormality or mild malocclusion	No or little need	≤ 25
Definite malocclusion	Elective	26 a 30
Severe malocclusion	Highly desirable	31 a 35
Very severe or disabling malocclusion	Essential	≥ 36

The examinations were carried out in a room in the school itself, under natural light, with the help of a clinical mirror and a millimeter periodontal probe

(The oral assessments were carried out by a single examiner after an intra-examiner calibration process. The records were recorded by a note-taker on a clinical epidemiological form (Appendices E and F), adapted from the World Health Organization (WHO, 1997).

3.8 Interview on self-perception

The schoolchildren were given a questionnaire in the form of a structured interview, which not only included questions about satisfaction with their appearance, but also made it possible to obtain information about their perception of the need for orthodontic treatment (Appendix G).

3.9 Pilot study

In order to test all the operational aspects, a pilot study was carried out involving 20 adolescents from a school that was not part of the main study. In addition to assessing logistical difficulties, this study allowed for the training and calibration of the examiner with a view to standardizing the use of the diagnostic criteria and allowed for the improvement of the collection tools. During the fieldwork, 10% of the sample was re-examined to check intra-examiner diagnostic agreement for each type of malocclusion, which was measured using the Kappa statistical test.

3.10 Statistical Data Analysis

At the same time as the data was collected, it was processed into a database. The statistical package Statistical Package for Social Science - SPSS (KINNEAR, 1997), version 15.0, was used, with a single entry, providing the research with greater reliability and trustworthiness.

Firstly, a descriptive analysis was carried out, obtaining the absolute and percentage distributions; the mean, median, standard deviation, minimum and maximum of each variable surveyed. For the association between the independent variables and the normative and self-perceived needs in relation to orthodontic treatment, a univariate analysis was used using the chi-square test (χ^2).

The Poisson regression model was used to measure the effect of exposure to the explanatory variables on the primary outcome (normative need for orthodontic treatment) and its magnitude was calculated using the Prevalence Ratio (PR), with a 95% confidence interval. In this procedure, the most significant results of the associations between the explanatory factors were selected for the initial model. This was used to check whether the addition of a particular factor would increase the model's ability to predict the need for orthodontic treatment. If the addition of a factor increased prediction, it remained in the model, and if not, it was rejected. This analysis was carried out using the Stata 9 statistical package (Stata Corp., version 9). Statistical significance was set at 5%.

Spearman's correlation was used to assess the relationship between the adolescent's visual analog scale and the professional's scale in relation to the need for orthodontic treatment.

In order to carry out the statistical analysis, the normative need for orthodontic treatment was dichotomized into two groups:

DAI score ≤ 30 - no need for treatment.

DAI score ≥ 31 - in need of treatment.

5. RESULTS

Of a total of 469 informed consent forms distributed to guardians, 431 were signed and 428 adolescents completed all stages of the survey (response rate = 91.7%). Intra-examiner agreement was high (Kappa between 0.8 and 1.0).

Table 1 shows their socio-demographic characterization. It can be seen that there was a predominance of females (67.1%) and 15-year-olds (36.0%). The average age of the sample was 16. As far as their mothers were concerned, they were on average 42 years old, with a few being over 49 (12.3%). They had little schooling (47.0%), with an average of 9 years of study. The average monthly family income was R$ 1500.00 (3.6 minimum wages).

TABLE 1 - Socio-demographic characteristics of high school students in Londrina - PR (N=428).

Behavior	N	%
Adolescent's gender		
Male	141	32,9
Female	287	67,1
Age of teenager		
15 years	154	36,0
16 years old	149	34,8
17 years old	103	24,1
18 years old	14	3,3
19 years old	8	1,9
Color		
White	272	63,6
Black	34	7,9
Brown	112	26,0
Yellow	10	2,3
Mother's age		
27-37 years	92	23,4
38-48 years	253	64,2
49 and over	49	12,4
Maternal Schooling		
0 to 8 years of schooling	185	47,0
9 to 11 years of schooling	144	36,5
12 and + years of study	65	16,5
Family Income (R$)		
0 - 1245,00	139	39,0
1246,00- 2075,00	112	31,5

| 2076,00 e + | 105 | 29,5 |

The prevalence of malocclusion found for the schoolchildren, according to the Angle classification, was 88.1% (Graph 1)

Graph 1. Classification of occlusion according to ANGLE

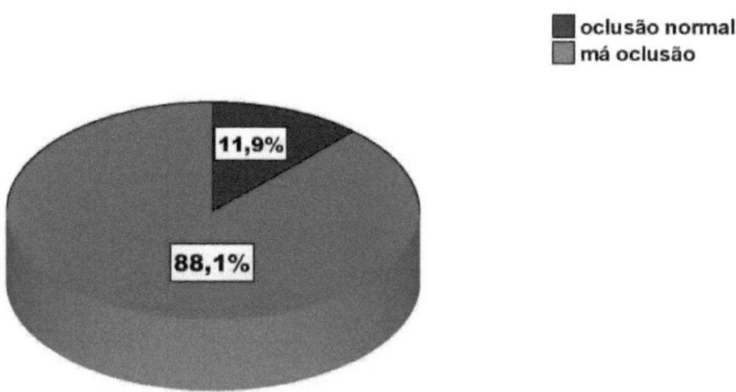

According to the normative criteria of the DAI index (Table 2), normal occlusion or the presence of mild malocclusion was detected in 72.6% of adolescents (no need for OT), while 13.7% had definite malocclusion (elective OT), 5.6% had severe malocclusion (highly desirable OT) and 7.4% had disabling malocclusion (fundamental OT). Overall, the normative need for orthodontic treatment was detected in 26.7% of schoolchildren. According to the cut-off point of 31 and the normative criteria of the DAI, orthodontic treatment was considered necessary in 56 individuals (13%).

The sensitivity and specificity of the index were not observed, especially in cases of mild or definite malocclusions, probably due to the divergence of criteria between the DAI index and the Angle classification.

As for the indicators of malocclusion in the DAI, dental crowding in one or two arches was the most prevalent (61.2%), followed by spacing in the anterior segment (18.0%), overjet greater than or equal to 4 mm (17.5%) and anterior open bite (7.0%). Median diastema greater than or equal to 2 mm (3.5%) and anterior crossbite (0.9%) were the least prevalent alterations (Table 2).

TABLE 2 - Distribution of DAI indicators of malocclusion and need for treatment for this pathology in 428 schoolchildren aged 15 to 19 in Londrina - PR .

	N	%
Molar ratio		
Class I	324	75,7
Class II or III	104	24,3

Anterior segment crowding		
Absent	166	38,8
1 or 2 arches	262	61,2
Anterior crowding		
< 2mm	391	91,4
> 2mm	37	8,6
Anterior lower crowding		
< 2mm	403	94,1
> 2mm	25	5,9
Overshoot		
< 4mm	353	82,5
> 4mm	75	17,5
Spacing in the anterior segment		
None	351	82,0
One or two segments	77	18,0
Median diastema		
< 2mm	413	96,5
> 2mm	15	3,5
Missing teeth		
None	390	91,1
One or more	38	8,9
Anterior open bite		
< 2mm	425	99,3
> 2mm	3	0,7
Anterior crossbite		
No	424	99,1
Yes	4	0,9
Need for orthodontic treatment		
No need	313	72,6
Elective	59	13,7
Highly desirable	24	5,6
Fundamental	32	7,4

As for the adolescents' perceptions (Table 3), the largest proportion of students (52.8%) said they were satisfied with the appearance of their teeth and their smiles (59.8%). However, 69.4% expressed a desire to improve their smiles and 75.7% to change them, 37.6% of whom wanted to change the position of their teeth. It's worth noting that a similar proportion of young people (55.1%) and their guardians (52.8%) reported the need for orthodontic treatment.

Despite the lack of statistical significance, the study of the association between socio-demographic variables and the normative need for orthodontic treatment (Table 4) showed that there was a higher indication of orthodontic treatment being highly desirable/mandatory among females (66.1%), white schoolchildren (63.5%), with mothers over 41 years of age (61.0%), with low schooling and belonging to a group of children with low education,1%), for the 15 to 16 age group (69.6%), among white schoolchildren (63.5), with mothers over 41 years old (61.0%), with low levels of schooling and belonging to families whose incomes were above 3 minimum wages (MW).

TABLE 3 - Perception of adolescents and their guardians regarding malocclusion and the need for treatment for this pathology in Londrina - PR .

	N	*%*
Satisfaction with the appearance of teeth		
Satisfied	226	52,8
Dissatisfied	202	47,2
Smile satisfaction		
Satisfied	256	59,8
Dissatisfied	172	40,2
How your oral health affects yours relationships with other people		
It doesn't affect	325	75,9
Affects	103	24,1
You'd like to improve your smile		
Yes	297	69,4
No	131	30,6
You'd like to change your smile		
Yes	324	75,7
No	104	24,3
What you would like to change		
Color	137	32,0
Size	26	6,1
Position	161	37,6
Nothing	104	24,3
You avoid smiling because of the way you look teeth		
Yes	128	29,9
No	300	70,1
You think you need orthodontic treatment		
Yes	236	55,1
No	192	44,9
Do you think your child needs treatment orthodontic		
Yes	200	52,8
No	179	47,2

TABLE 4 - Normative need for orthodontic treatment (DAI) of adolescents from Londrina - PR,

according to socio-demographic characteristics (N=428).

Features	No need		In need		Value of
		from TO		from TO	p
	N	%	N	%	
Adolescent's gender					
Male	102	32,6	39	33,9	
Female	211	67,4	76	66,1	0,796
Age of teenager					
15 to 16 years old	223	71,2	80	69,6	
17 to 19 years old	90	28,8	35	30,4	0,735
Skin color					
White	199	63,6	73	63,5	
Other	114	36,4	42	36,5	0,985
Mother's age					
28 to 40 years old	128	44,3	41	39,0	
Over 41	161	55,7	64	61,0	0,353
Maternal Schooling					
0 to 8 years of schooling	130	44,8	55	52,9	
Over 9 years of schooling	160	55,2	49	47,1	0,158
Family Income (R$)					
Up to 3 MW	100	38,3	39	41,1	
Above 3 MW	161	61,7	56	58,9	0,640

Chi-square test; n.s.

Table 5 shows the results of the univariate analyses for the dependent variable "need for normative treatment", according to the self-perception of the adolescents, their guardians and the use of orthodontic braces. Adolescents who were dissatisfied with the appearance of their teeth and their smile, and who wanted to improve their smile, represented the largest proportion of the population in need of orthodontic treatment, as evidenced by the statistical association. Of the adolescents in need of orthodontic treatment, 77.4% believed they needed it, an opinion shared by 73.3% of guardians. It is worth noting that 41.7% of the schoolchildren were undergoing orthodontic treatment or had already finished it.

TABLE 5 - Normative need for TO among adolescents in Londrina - PR, according to their self-perception, that of their guardians and the use of orthodontic braces (N=428).

	No need (DAI) N%		With need N%		(DAI)P
Satisfaction with the appearance of teeth					
Satisfied	182	58,1	44	38,3	
Dissatisfied	131	41,9	71	61,7	0,000***
Smile satisfaction					

Satisfied	206	65,8	50	43,5	
Dissatisfied	107	34,2	65	56,5	0,000***
Avoids smiling due to the appearance of your teeth					
Yes	81	25,9	47	40,9	
No	232	74,1	68	59,1	0,003**
Would you like to improve your smile					
Yes	201	64,2	96	83,5	
No	112	35,8	19	16,5	0,000***
Do you think you need TO					
Yes	147	47,0	89	77,4	
No	166	53,0	26	22,6	0,000***
Responsible person's perception of need for TO					
Yes	123	44,9	77	73,3	
No	151	55,1	28	26,7	0,000***
You wear or have worn braces orthodontic					
Yes	117	37,4	48	41,7	
No	196	62,6	67	58,3	0,412

Chi-square test; **p<0.01,***p<0.001

Table 6 shows the results of the univariate analyses between the dependent variable "self-perceived need for treatment" (subjective criterion), the indicators of malocclusion (components of the DAI), the prevalence of malocclusion and the normative need for OT. Among the components of the DAI, the following showed a significant association: presence of incisal crowding greater than 2 mm, overjet of 4 mm or more and missing teeth. On the other hand, anterior open bite, anterior crossbite, anterior segment spacing and median diastema were not statistically associated with the adolescent's perception of the need for orthodontic treatment. It is worth noting that self-perceived need was also associated with the prevalence of malocclusion (p=0.029).

Although there was a significant association between normative and self-perceived orthodontic treatment needs, the high number of schoolchildren (86.5%) who declared the need for orthodontic treatment, classified by the DAI as not needing it, is noteworthy (Table 6).

The univariate analysis of the dependent variable "satisfaction with appearance" (subjective criterion) and the normative criteria showed no association with median diastema, missing teeth, anterior open bite and anterior crossbite (Table 7). On the contrary, there was a statistical association with anterior crowding in one or both arches, overjet and anterior spacing.

TABLE 6 - Self-perceived need for orthodontic treatment (OT) among adolescents in Londrina - PR, according to malocclusion indicators and the DAI classification (N=428).

	No need		In need		*P*
	N	**%**	**N**	**%**	
Molar ratio					
Class I	169	71,6	155	80,7	
Class II or III	67	28,4	37	19,3	0,029*
Anterior segment crowding					
Absent	72	30,5	94	40,9	
1 or 2 arches	164	69,5	98	51,0	0,000***
Anterior crowding					
< 2mm	204	86,4	187	97,4	
> 2mm	32	13,6	5	2,6	0,000***
Anterior lower crowding					
< 2mm	214	90,7	188	98,4	
> 2mm	22	9,3	3	1,6	0,001***
Over-emphasis					
< 4mm	185	78,4	168	87,5	
> 4mm	51	21,6	24	12,5	0,014*
Spacing in the anterior segment					
None	188	79,7	163	84,9	
One or two segments	48	20,3	29	15,1	0,161
Median diastema					
< 2mm	225	95,3	188	97,9	
> 2mm	11	4,7	4	2,1	0,150
Missing teeth					
None	207	87,7	183	95,3	
One or more	29	12,3	9	4,7	0,006**
Anterior open bite					
< 2mm	234	99,2	191	99,5	
> 2mm	2	0,8	1	0,5	0,987
Anterior crossbite					
No	233	98,7	191	99,5	
Yes	3	1,3	1	0,5	0,423
Need for orthodontic treatment					
No need	147	62,3	166	86,5	
Elective	43	18,2	16	8,3	
Highly desirable	20	8,5	4	2,1	

| Fundamental | 26 | 11,0 | 6 | 3,1 | 0,000*** |

Chi-square test; *p<0.05,**p<0.01,***p<0.001

TABLE 7 - Association between malocclusion indicators and satisfaction with the appearance of teeth in 428 schoolchildren aged 15 to 19 in Londrina - PR

	Satisfied		Dissatisfied		P
	N	**%**	**N**	**%**	
Molar ratio					
Class I	179	79,2	145	71,8	
Class II or III	47	20,8	57	28,2	0,074
Anterior segment crowding					
Absent	101	44,7	65	32,2	
1 or 2 arches	125	55,3	137	67,8	0,008**
Anterior crowding					
< 2mm	218	96,5	173	85,6	
> 2mm	8	3,5	29	14,4	0,000***
Anterior lower crowding					
< 2mm	219	97,3	183	90,6	
> 2mm	6	2,7	19	9,4	0,003**
Over-emphasis					
< 4mm	197	87,2	156	77,2	
> 4mm	29	12,8	46	22,8	0,007**
Spacing in the anterior segment					
None	195	86,3	156	77,2	
One or two segments	31	13,7	46	22,8	0,015*
Median diastema					
< 2mm	220	97,3	193	95,5	
> 2mm	6	2,7	9	4,5	0,312
Missing teeth					
None	208	92,0	182	90,1	
One or more	18	8,0	20	9,9	0,483
Anterior open bite					
< 2mm	225	99,6	200	99,0	
> 2mm	1	4,0	2	1,0	0,498
Anterior crossbite					
No	225	99,6	199	98,5	
Yes	1	4,0	3	1,5	0,264

Chi-square test; *p<0.05,**p<0.01,***p<0.001

Chi-square analysis showed that adolescents who lived in the central region of Londrina, were dissatisfied with the appearance of their teeth and smile, who said they avoided smiling and expressed a desire to change it were more associated with the need for TO according to normative criteria (Tables 8 and 9).

After univariate analysis, only two variables were statistically significant using Poisson regression: satisfaction with the smile (PR=1.64; 95%CI: 1.05-2.56) and studying in the central region (PR=0.18; 95%CI: 0.40-0.86) (Table 10).

There was a moderate correlation (r= 0.61) between the adolescent's visual analogue scale and that of the professional in relation to the need for orthodontic treatment.

TABLE 8 - Univariate analysis of socio-demographic factors related to the normative need for orthodontic treatment

Variable	X^2	P
Gender	0,020	0,88
Age	0,048	0,82
Skin color	0,000	1,00
Maternal age	0,665	0,41
Maternal education	0,168	0,19
Family Income	0,119	0,73
Region	16,94	0,002*

TABLE 9 - Univariate analysis of the questions relating to adolescents' perceptions of the normative need for TO

Variable	X^2	P
Adolescents' satisfaction with the appearance of their teeth	12,55	0,001*
Adolescent satisfaction with their smile	16,53	0,001*
Oral health interfering with relationships	2,20	0,137
Avoid smiling	8,31	0,004*
I'd like to change my smile	13,79	0,001*
I use braces	0,503	0,47

TABLE 10 - Multivariate analysis of the two main factors related to the normative need for orthodontic treatment

Variable	Estimate	Standard Error	P	PR (95% CI)
Central Region	1,67	0,78	0,03	0,18 (0,40;0,86)
Satisfaction with a smile	5,49	1,23	<0,001	1,64 (1,05;2,56)

PR: Prevalence Ratio; CI: Confidence Interval;

6. DISCUSSION

Since the end of the 19th century, various classification systems have been proposed by different authors, initially with the aim of facilitating orthodontic diagnosis and treatment, and later to serve efficiently and accurately for epidemiological studies. Angle's classification (ARAÙJO, 1986) became the main instrument for measuring malocclusions throughout the last century. Due to its limitations, both in assessing malocclusions in the vertical and transverse directions and due to the lack of criteria needed to be considered an epidemiological instrument, various authors have proposed other systems to replace Angle's system, but none of them have been widely used. Since 1997, the World Health Organization (WHO) has recommended the use of a quantitative record to assess malocclusion (PINTO et al. 2008), using the dental aesthetic index (DAI). The population in this study was assessed using both malocclusion classification methods.

The high response rate and good intra-examiner agreement for the malocclusions studied provide consistency and credibility to the results.

The prevalence of malocclusion in the population studied, according to Angle's classification, was 88.3%, a result similar to that found by Silva Filho et al. in 1989 (88.5%), Peres et al. in 2002 (71.3%), Onyeaso in 2004 (76%), and to a lesser extent by Perin in 2002 (66.7%) and Marques in 2005 (61.9%).

At least one type of malocclusion was observed in 24.3% of the participants using the DAI. This figure is similar to those found in studies carried out with adolescents in Brazil, such as in São Paulo (REYES et al. 2002; JAHN,2005) and contrary to the studies carried out by Peres et al, 2002; Marques et al. 2005; Santos (2006); Moura (2007); Peres et al. (2008) and the national survey (SB2004), The differences may have been due to the method used to select the sample and the criteria used for diagnosis.

There was no difference between the genders in the distribution of malocclusion according to the DAI, similar to the results of Jahn (2005) and Onyeaso et al. (2005), unlike Peres et al. 2002 and Moura (2007), who observed a higher prevalence in males.

The most prevalent types of malocclusion were dental crowding in one or two segments (61.2%), overjet equal to or greater than 4mm (17.5%), consistent with the results of Marques et al. 2005; Peres et al. 2005 and Santos,2006 and spacing in the anterior teeth (18.0%), lower than the values found by Marques et al. 2005. Since facial aesthetics is considered an important factor in terms of society's and individuals' perceptions and concepts of themselves, it is worth emphasizing the relationship between the overjet, crowding and spacing components and the self-perception of the need for treatment found in this study.

Values for median diastema equal to or greater than 2mm (2.1%), anterior spacing of one or two segments (15.1%), anterior open bite greater than or equal to 2mm (0.5%) and anterior crossbite (0.5%) corroborated the studies carried out by Santos (2006) and showed no statistically significant association with self-perceived need for treatment.

Adolescents with crowding in one or more segments were more dissatisfied with their dental appearance, regardless of any other malocclusion, which corroborates the studies by MARQUES et al. (2005), PERES et al. (2002).

Parents' desire for orthodontic treatment for their children was lower than that of adolescents, contrary to studies by Hamdan (2004).

Establishing the anteroposterior molar ratio can be flawed, especially when the assessment is carried out directly in the mouth, as in our study. Attention should therefore be paid to determining this component, considering that it has a weight of 3 (SANTOS, 2006). Despite the importance of the molar ratio for diagnosis, 71.8% of schoolchildren with normal occlusion (DAI) said they were dissatisfied with the appearance of their teeth, emphasizing the importance of aesthetic aspects in personal satisfaction. Orthodontic problems in the region of the posterior teeth do not seem to have an impact on satisfaction with appearance, nor on the need for treatment perceived by individuals (SHAW et al. 1975). However, we should not underestimate the presence of occlusal interferences as a possible etiological factor in temporomandibular disorders.

Occlusion problems such as posterior crossbite, posterior open bite, deep bite, midline deviation, dental impactions and missing molars are not verified in the DAI (DANYLUK et al.1999). These factors can have a considerable impact on the diagnosis of orthodontic treatment needs, which could jeopardize the validity of the index (PERIN, 2000), as they showed a moderate prevalence when assessed by Silva Filho et al (1989), with 18.2% of posterior crossbite and 19.8% of deep bite, according to Angle's classification.

The need for orthodontic treatment is not always easily defined by the professional, perhaps because deviations from normal occlusion are not always clear and easy to identify; in other words, it is difficult to delineate acceptable and unacceptable occlusions. Therefore, the indication for treatment can be better defined by the professional with the addition of other tests, occlusal normative indices and knowledge of the existence of the negative impact of malocclusion on the individual's quality of life (MARQUES et al. 2005).

Through the use of the Dental Aesthetics Index (DAI), the World Health Organization has tried to establish a simple, universally accepted method that can be used in epidemiological surveys to establish the need for orthodontic treatment and the priority of orthodontic care in public programs. Despite being objective, simple and easy to apply, it was not sensitive to some occlusal problems, which could be confirmed by the results obtained in this study, especially in cases where elective treatment was needed, corroborating the studies by Reyes et al, 2004. The discrepancy between the prevalence values of malocclusion found using the DAI and the Angle classification is evident, showing that the former only partially covers occlusal problems and should be reviewed and modified as a tool for assessing malocclusion in public health. The same difference was found by Perin in 2002, who found 66.7% of malocclusion using Angle and 34.7% using the DAI.

Turner, in 1990, emphasized the difficulty of classifying malocclusion in epidemiology and of creating an index that covered all aspects of malocclusion and that could be used consistently by non-orthodontically trained personnel. Similarly, Bresolin in 2000 considered the creation of indices representative of the different degrees of severity of malocclusion to be a real challenge.

It seems valid to suggest including the items posterior crossbite and/or posterior open bite and/or deep bite in the DAI clinical examination form, in order to minimize its limitations. We should also not overlook the fact that both indices do not assess and diagnose temporomandibular disorders. Furthermore, it is worth pointing out that the etiology of some malocclusion descriptors (anterior open bite, Class II or III molar relationship, among others) can be different for the same value obtained from the DAI, as they are often problems of dental, skeletal and/or functional origin, which require different therapeutic approaches.

Once the suggested modifications are adopted, the index could be used by dental hygienists to determine which patients to refer to specialists, which could cut down on a large number of initial consultations by dentists and orthodontists, an important advantage in public health programs. In addition, DAI scores have been significantly associated with the perception of the need for treatment by students and guardians, and are good predictors of the acceptance of future corrective orthodontic treatment (ONYEASO and SANU, 2005). Orthodontic treatment is not routinely offered in Brazilian public dental services. Due to the scarcity of treatment, DAI can help dentists and health managers develop strategies to provide equal access to orthodontic treatment, meeting the treatment needs of the population.

7. CONCLUSIONS

From the results obtained in this study, it can be concluded that:

> The prevalence of malocclusion found in the schoolchildren was 26.7% according to the DAI and 88.1% using the Angle classification.

> According to the DAI, severe, very severe or disabling malocclusions with great need or mandatory need for orthodontic treatment were found in 13.0% of the sample.

> Regarding the perception of the need for orthodontic treatment by adolescents and their guardians, 55.1% and 53.1% were found, respectively.

> The socio-demographic factors studied showed no statistically significant association with normative and self-perceived orthodontic treatment needs.

> Dissatisfaction with appearance was a predictor of normative need for treatment, while the central region was a protective factor.

> There was a moderate correlation (r= 0.61) between the adolescent's visual analogue scale and that of the professional in relation to the need for orthodontic treatment.

When assessing the degree of need for orthodontic treatment of adolescents, following the occlusal assessment parameters routinely used by orthodontists (Angle classification), the vast majority showed a need for treatment. If occlusal indices could be adopted, especially in the public network, when assessing the need for orthodontic treatment, almost all of the vacancies would be channeled towards the most severe cases.

Occlusal indices represent data collection tools from an epidemiological point of view. The IOTN and DAI indices are not a substitute for diagnosis and case planning and do not allow orthodontists to do without orthodontic documentation.

8. REFERENCES

ARAÙJO, M. C. Malocclusions: classification of malocclusions: description of dental malpositions. In: . **Orthodontics for clinicians**. 3. ed. Sâo Paulo: Ed. Santos, 1986. Chap.4, p. 99-107.

BACA-GARCIA, A. et al. Malocclusions and orthodontic treatment needs in a group of Spanish adolescents using the Dental Aesthetic Index. **Int Dent J**, London, v.54, n.3, p. 139-142, 2004.

BARBETTA, P.A. **Estatistica aplicada às ciências sociais**. Florianopolis. ed. da UFSC, 2007, 315 p.

BAUME, L. J. Uniform methods for the epidemiologic assessment of malocclusion: results obtained with the World Health Organization standard methods (1962 and 1971) in South Pacific populations. **Am. J. Orthod.**, St. Louis, MO, v. 66, n. 3, p. 251-272, sep. 1974.

BELL, R. et al. Perceptions of facial profile and their influence on the decision to undergo orthognatic surgery. **Am. J. Orthod. Dentofacial Orthop.**, St. Louis, MO, n. 88, p. 323-332, Oct. 1985.

BRAZIL. Ministry of Health. National Oral Health Coordination. **SB Brasil Project:** oral health conditions of the Brazilian population 2002-2003: main results. Brasilia, 2004b.

BRAZIL. Ministry of Health. Health Programs. **Smiling Brazil.** Available at: http://portal.saude.gov.br/portal/saùde. Accessed on: 28 Feb 2008.

BRESOLIN, D. malocclusion indices. In: Pinto VG, organizer. **Collective oral health.** Sâo Paulo: Editora Santos;. p. 197-302, 2000.

BROOK, P. H.; SHAW, W. C. The development of an index of orthodontic treatment priority. **Eur. J. Orthod.**, London, v. 11, n. 3, p. 309-320, aug. 1989.

COOPER, S. et al. The reliability of the index of orthodontic treatment need over time. **Journal of Orthodontics**, Manchester, U.K., v. 27, n.1; p.47-53, mar. 2000.

CONS, N. C. et al. Perceptions of occlusal conditions in Australia, the German Democratic Republic and the United States of America. **Int. Dent. J.**, London, v. 33; p. 200-206, 1983.

CONS, N.; JENNY, J.; KOHOUT, F. **DAI**: The Dental Aesthetic Index. Iowa City: College of Dentistry, University of Iowa, 1986.

CUNHA, A.; MIGUEL, J.; LIMA, K. Evaluation of the DAI and IOTN indices in the diagnosis of malocclusions and the need for orthodontic treatment. **Rev. Dental Press Ortodon.**

Orthop. Facial, Maringà, PR, v. 8, n. 1, p. 51-58, ,jan./feb. 2003.

DANYLUK, K.; LAVELLE, C.; HASSARD, T. Potential application of the dental aesthetic index to prioritize the orthodontic service needs in a publicly funded dental program. **Am J Orthod Dentofacial Orthop,** St. Louis, MO , v.116, n.3, p.279-86, sep 1999.

DIAS, P.; GLEISER, R. The orthodontic treatment needs index as a public health evaluation method. **R. Dental Press Ortodon. Orthop. Facial**, Maringà, PR, v. 13, n. 1, p. 74-81, jan./feb. 2008.

ESPELAND, L. et al. Perception of malocclusion in 11-year-old children: a comparison between personal and parental awareness. **Eur. J. Orthod.,** London, v. 14, n. 5, p. 350-358, Oct. 1992.

FRAZÂO, P.; NARVAI, P. Socio-environmental Factors Associated with Dental Occlusion in Adolescents. **Am J Orthod Dentofacial Orthop,** St. Louis, MO, v.129, n.6, p.809-16, 2006.

GALVÂO, C.; PEREIRA, C.; BELLO, D. Prevalence of malocclusions in Latin America and anthropological considerations. **Ortodontia** v.27; p. 52-59, 1994.

GHERUNPONG, S.; TSAKOS, G.; SHEIHAM, A. A socio-dental approach to assessing children's orthodontic needs. **Eur. J. Orthod.,** London, v. 28, p. 393-399, May 2006.

GRZYWACZ, I. The value of the aesthetic component of the index of orthodontic treatment need in the assessment of subjective orthodontic treatment need. **Eur. J. Orthod.,** London, v. 25, p. 57-63, 2003.

HAMDAN, A. The relationship between patient, parent and clinician perceived need and normative orthodontic treatment need. **Eur. J. Orthod.,** London, v. 26, p. 265271,2004.

HANCOCK, P. A.; BLINKHORN, A. S. A comparison of the perceived and normative needs for dental care in 12 year-old children in the northwest of England. **Community Dent. Health,** London, v. 13, p. 81-85, 1996.

HUNT, O. et al. The aesthetic component of the index of orthodontic treatment need validates against lay opinion. **Eur. J. Orthod.,** London, v. 24, p. 53-59, 2002.

BRAZILIAN INSTITUTE OF GEOGRAPHY AND STATISTICS. IBGE **cidades@.** 2006. Available at: http://www.ibge.gov.br/cidadesat/default.php. Accessed on: March 24, 2008.

JAHN, G. **Dental occlusion in schoolchildren and adolescents in the state of Sao Paulo.** 2002. Dissertation (Master's Degree in Dentistry) - USP School of Dentistry, Sao Paulo, 2005.

JENNY, J; CONS, N. C. Comparing and contrasting two orthodontics indices, the Index of Orthodontic Treatment Need and the Dental Aesthetic Index. **Am J Orthod Dentofacial Orthop,** St. Louis, MO, v.110, n.4, p. 410-416, 1996.

JOHANSSON, A.; FOLLIN, M. Evaluation of the aesthetic component of the Index of Orthodontic Treatment Need by Swedish orthodontists. **Eur. J. Orthod.**, London, v. 27, p. 160-166, 2005.

KEROSUO, H. et al. The influence of incisal malocclusion on the social attractiveness of young people in Finland. **Eur. J. Orthod.**, London, v. 17, p. 505-512, 1995.

KINNEAR, P. R.; GRAY, C. D. **SPSS for windows, made simple.** 2. ed. New York: Psychology Press, 1997.

KOOCHEK, A.; SHUE-TE YEH, M.; RICHMOND, S. The relationship between index of complexity, outcome and need, and patient's perceptions of malocclusion: a study in general dental practice. **Br. Dent. J.**, London, v. 191, n. 6, p.325-329, Sept. 2001.

LOW, W.; TAN, S.; SCHWARZ, S. The effect of severe caries on the quality of life in young children. **Pediatr. Dent.,** Chicago, IL, v. 21, n. 6, p. 325-326, 1999.

MANDALL, N. et al. Perceived aesthetic impact of malocclusion and oral self-perceptions in 14-15-year-old Asian and Caucasian children in Greater Manchester. **Eur. J. Orthod.**, London, n. 21, p. 175-183, 1999.

MARQUES, L. et al. Prevalence of malocclusion and need for orthodontic treatment in schoolchildren aged 10 to 14 years in Belo Horizonte, Minas Gerais, Brazil: a psychosocial approach. **Cad. Saùde Pùblica**, Rio de Janeiro, v. 21, n. 4, p. 1099-1106, jul./ago. 2005.

. Malocclusion: Esthetic impact and quality of life among Brazilian schoolchildren. **Am. J. Orthod. Dent. Orthop.**, St. Louis, MO, v. 129, n. 3, p. 424427, mar. 2006.

MOURA, C.; CAVALCANTI, A. Malocclusions, dental caries and perceptions of aesthetics and masticatory function: an association study. **Rev. Odonto Ciência**, Porto Alegre, v. 22, n. 57, jul./set. 2007.

MOYERS, R. E. Classification and terminology of malocclusion. In: . **Orthodontics.** 4. ed. Rio de Janeiro: Guanabara Koogan, 1991. ch. 9, p. 156-166.

NASH, D. Professional ethics and esthetic dentistry. **J. Am. Dent. Assoc.**, Chicago, Ill., Special Issue,7-9-E, Sept. 1988.

OLIVEIRA, C. M. de. Malocclusion in the context of public health. In: BONECkER, M.;

SHEIHAM, A. **Promoting oral health in childhood and adolescence**: knowledge and practices. Sao Paulo: Santos, 2004. ch. 4, p. 55-80.

OLIVEIRA, C. M. de; SHEIHAM, A. The relationship between normative orthodontic treatment need and oral health-related quality of life. **Community Dent. Oral Epidemiol.**, Copenhagen, DK, v. 31, n. 6, p. 426-436, Dec. 2003.

ONYEASO, C. Prevalence of malocclusion among adolescents in Ibadan, Nigeria. **Am J Orthod Dentofacial Orthop**, St. Louis, MO, v.126, n.5, p. 604-607, nov 2004.

ONYEASO, C; SANU, O. Perception of personal dental appearance in Nigerian adolescents. **Am J Orthod Dentofacial Orthop**, St. Louis, Mo, v.127, n.6, p. 700706, 2005.

WORLD HEALTH ORGANIZATION. **Health through oral health; guidelines for planning and monitoring for oral health care. World Health Organization and Federation Dentaire Internationale.** London: Quintessence, 1989.

WORLD HEALTH ORGANIZATION. **Epidemiological survey of oral health**: instruction manual. 4. ed. Geneva: WHO, 1997.

PATEL, R.; TOOTLA, R.; INGLEHART, M. Does oral health affect self perceptions, parental ratings and video-based assesment of children's smiles? **Community Dent. Oral Epidemiol.,** Copenhagen, DK, v. 35, p. 44-52, 2007.

PERES, K. G.; TOMITA, N. E. Occlusopathies. In: ANTUNES, J. L. F.; PERES, M. A. **Fundamentals of dentistry**: epidemiology of oral health. Rio de Janeiro: Guanabara Koogan, 2006. p. 83-101.

PERES, K. G.; TRAEBERT, E.; MARCENES, W. Differences between self-perception and normative criteria in the identification of malocclusions. **Rev. Saùde Pùblica**, Sao Paulo, v. 36, n. 2, p. 230-236, 2002.

PERES, K. G. et al. Does malocclusion influence the adolescent's satisfaction with appearance? A cross-sectional study nested in a Brazilian birth cohort. **Community Dent. Oral Epidemiol.**, Copenhagen, DK, v. 36, p. 137-143, 2008.

PERIN, Paulo César Pereira. **Prevalence of malocclusion and need for orthodontic treatment, comparing the Angle classification and the dental esthetics index, in the city of Lins/SP.** 2002. Thesis (Doctorate) - Araçatuba School of Dentistry. Universidade Estadual Paulista, Araçatuba, SP, 2002.

PHILIPS, C.; GRIFFIN, T.; BENNETT, E. Perception of facial attractiveness by patients, peers, and professionals. **Int. J. Adult Orthodon. Orthognath Surg.**, Chicago, ILL, v. 10, p. 127-135, 1995.

PINHEIRO, F. et al. Comparison of the perception and esthetic need for orthodontic treatment between patients and orthodontists in the cities of Natal/RN and Joâo Pessoa/PB. **Rev. Dental Press Ortodon. Orthop. Facial,** Maringà, PR, v. 10, n. 2, p. 54-61, mar./abr. 2005.

PINTO, S. Determining dental treatment needs: A social approach. **Saùde Bucal Coletiva**. 4. ed. Sâo Paulo: Santos, 2000. chap. 6, p. 223-250.

PINTO, E.; GONDIM, P.; LIMA, N. Critical analysis of the various methods for evaluating and recording malocclusions. **Rev. Dental Press Ortodon. Orthop. Facial,** Maringà, PR, v. 13, n. 1, p. 82-91, jan./feb. 2008.

PROFFIT, W. R.; FIELDS JR., H. W. **Contemporary orthodontics**. Rio de Janeiro: Guanabara Koogan, 1995. p. 2-15.

REIS, H.; WILSON, I.; MONESTER, C. What is smiling is beautiful and good. **Eur. J. Soc. Psychol.** The Hague, n. 20, p. 259-267, 1990.

REYES,L et al. Malocclusions by the dental esthetic index (DAI) in the under-19 population. **Rev cubana Estomatol,** Ciudad de La Habana, v.41, n.3, sept- dec., 2004.

SALZMANN, J. A. Handicapping malocclusin assessment to establish treatment priority. **Am. J. Orthod.,** St. Louis, MO, v. 54, n. 10, p. 749-765, 1968.

SANDY, J.; ROBERTS-HARRY, D. **A clinical guideline to orthodontics**. London: British Dental Association, 2003.

SANTOS, P. C. F. dos. **Study of the prevalence of malocclusions and the need for treatment in patients at the integrated clinic of the School of Dentistry of the University of São Paulo**. 2006. Dissertation (Master's Degree in Dentistry) - University of São Paulo, São Paulo, 2006.

SHAW, W. C. et al. Quality control in orthodontics: risk/benefit consideration. **Br. Dent. J.,** London, v. 170, n. 1, p. 33-37, Jan. 1991.

SHAW, W. C.; LEWIS, H. G.; ROBERTSON, N. Perception of malocclusion. **Br. Dent. J.,** London, v. 138, n. 6, p. 211-216, Mar. 1975.

SHAW, W.; RICHMOND, S.; O'BRIEN, K. The use of occlusal indices: a european perspective. **Am. J. Orthod. Dentofacial. Orthop.,** St. Louis, MO, v. 107, n. 1, p. 1-10, Jan. 1995.

SHEIHAM, A. Determining dental treatment needs: a social approach. In: PINTO, V. G. **Saùde bucal coletiva.** 4. ed. 2000.Sâo Paulo: Ed. Santos, 2000. Chap. 6, p. 223-250.

SHEIHAM, A.; MAIZELS, J.; MAIZELS, A. New composite indicators of dental health. **Community Dent. Health**, London, v. 4, n. 4, p. 407-414, Dec. 1987.

SILVA FILHO, O; FREITAS,S.; CAVASSAN,A. Prevalence of normal occlusion and malocclusion in the mixed dentition in schoolchildren in the city of Bauru (São Paulo). **Rev. Assoc. Paul. Cir. Dent.**; Sâo Paulo, v.43, n.6, p. 287-290, Nov-Dec. 1989.

SIMOES, W. A. Prevention of malocclusions. **Ortodontia**, Sâo Paulo, v. 11, p. 117125, 1978.

SLADE, G. D.; SPENCER, A. J. Development and evaluation of the oral health impact profile. **Community Dent. Health**, London, v. 11, n. 1, p. 3-11, Mar. 1994.

STENVICK, A. et al. Lay attitudes to dental appeal and need for orthodontic treatment. **Eur. J. Orthod.**, London, n. 19, p. 271-277, 1997.

TEDESCO, L. et al. A dento-facial attractiveness scale. Part I: reliability and validity. **Am. J. Orthod.**, St. Louis, MO, v. 83, n. 1, p. 38-46, 1983.

TURNER, S. Occlusal Indices revisited. **Br J Orthod**, London, n.17, p. 197-203, 1990.

9. ANNEXES

ANNEX A

Ethics Committee opinion

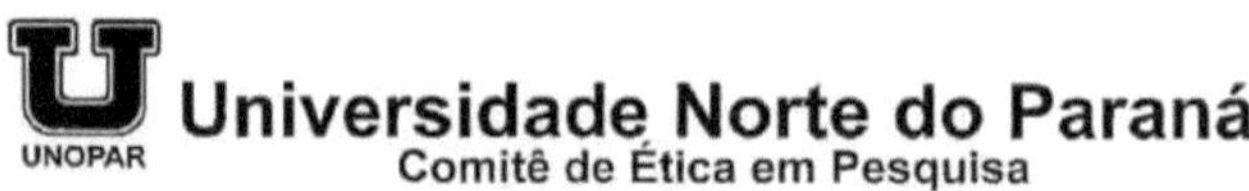

Universidade Norte do Paraná
Comitê de Ética em Pesquisa

CONSUBSTANTIATED OPINION

PROTOCOL: PP 0012/08

RESPONSIBLE: *Sandra Mara Maciel*

Unopar's Research Ethics Committee analyzed and APPROVED the ethical aspect of the project *"Study on genetic and behavioral risk factors common to dental caries and obesity in adolescents"*.

0 CEP/UNOPAR establishes:

a)   0 research subjects have the freedom to refuse to participate or to withdraw their consent at any stage of the research, without any penalty and without prejudice to their care (CNS Res. 196/96 - Item IV.1.f) and must receive a copy of the Free and Informed Consent Form, in its entirety, signed by them (Item IV.2.d).

b)   The researcher must carry out the research as outlined in the approved protocol and discontinue the study only after analysis of the reasons for discontinuation by CEP/UNOPAR (CNS Res Item III.3.z), awaiting its opinion, except when he/she perceives unanticipated risk or harm to the subject or when he/she verifies the Superiority of the Regimen Offered to one of the research groups (Item V.3) that require immediate action.

c)   O CEP/UNOPAR must be informed of all adverse effects or relevant facts that alter the normal course of the study (CNS Res. Item V.4). It is the researcher's role to ensure that appropriate measures are taken immediately in the event of a serious adverse event (even if it occurred at another center) and to send notification to CEP/UNOPAR together with their position.

d)   Any modifications or amendments to the protocol must be presented to CEP/UNOPAR in a clear and succinct manner, identifying the part of the protocol to be modified and its justifications.

e)   Partial reports must be submitted every six months and the final report at the end of the project.

Londrina, May 09, 2008

Prof. Dr. Hélr/tjÿstii Suguimoto President dC^z C.EP. UNOPAR

ANNEX B

Letter of Authorization from the Regional Education Center

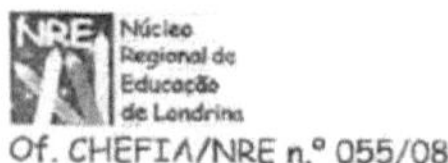

Of. CHEFIA/NRE n.º 055/08

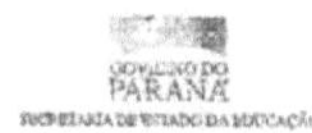

Londrina, 31 de janeiro de 2008.

Dear Madam

We would like to thank Your Excellency's SoIicitacSo for authorizing the collection of data to carry out the researches "Comparison between norm Hvas needs for orthodontic treatment and self-perceived needs in relation to malocclusion by adolescents from

Lendrina-PR" and "Studies on genetic and behavioral risk factors for dental caries and obesity in adolescents".

We enclose a copy of the list of state schools, by region, to facilitate access and obtain authorization from the school boards that may be selected for the data collection.

Sincerely

Márcia Maria Lopes de Souza
Chefe do NRE/LONDRINA
Decreto nº 743/07

lima Mrs

Prof.ª . Dr.ª Sandra AAara AAaciel

UNOPAR

Londrina - PR

ANNEX C

Research authorization

AUTHORIZATION

I authorize the research *"Comparison between normative needs for orthodontic treatment and self-perceived needs in relation to malocclusion by adolescents from Londrina-Pr"* and *"Studies on common risk factors for dental caries and obesity in adolescents"*, with high school students from Escola Polivalente de Londrina.

Profª. Maria Elizabeth Penteriche
Diretora

AUTHORIZATION

I authorize the research *"Comparison between normative needs for orthodontic treatment and self-perceived needs in relation to malocclusion by adolescents in Londrina-Pr. "* and *"Studies on common risk factors for dental caries and obesity in adolescents"*, with secondary school students at the Colégio Estadual Prof. Paulo Freire - Elementary and Secondary School.

Lourdes Mendes dos Santos
Diretora

ANNEX D

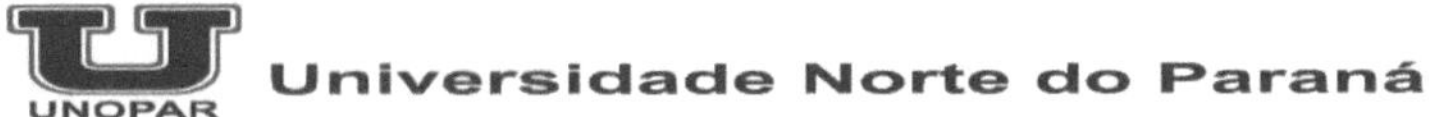

RESEARCH: COMPARISON BETWEEN NORMATIVE ORTHODONTIC TREATMENT NEEDS AND SELF-PERCEIVED NEEDS BY ADOLESCENTS IN LONDRINA-PR

INFORMATION LETTER TO THE PERSON RESPONSIBLE

Dear mother/father:

Unopar, through its Master's Degree in Dentistry, intends to carry out some research among adolescents aged between 15 and 19, enrolled in state schools. The research will be useful so that, at a later stage, actions can be planned and developed to guide dental professionals in their decision to treat adolescents orthodontically.

To this end, procedures will be adopted that have already been widely used in previous research/studies and have proven to be completely safe. In short, they will be carried out:

- clinical examination of adolescents' mouths: to check the condition of their teeth;

- the application of an interview with adolescents: to assess their perceptions of smile aesthetics.

- the formulation of a question to parents to assess their perception of the need for orthodontic treatment for their children.

The participant will be guaranteed: to receive answers to any questions or clarification of any doubts about the procedures, risks, benefits and other issues related to the research; the freedom to withdraw their consent at any time and stop participating in the study, without any prejudice; the security that they will not be identified and that the confidential nature of the information related to their privacy will be maintained.

INFORMED CONSENT FORM

By this instrument, which complies with legal requirements, Mr. ______________________

_______, bearer of identity card no. ______________________________________, after carefully reading the **INFORMATION LETTER TO THE RESPONSIBLE PARTY**, duly explained in detail by the professional, aware of the procedures to which your child will be subjected, leaving no doubts about what has been read and explained, signs your **FREE AND INFORMED CONSENT**, agreeing to participate in the proposed research.

In agreement, they sign this agreement.

In agreement, they sign this agreement.

_____________________________ _____________________________

Signature of responsible person Signature of researcher

Londrina, ____ of _________ of ______

ANNEX E

DAI

☐ ☐   DENTITION- number of I, C and PM lost

<u>SPACE*</u>

<table>
<tr><td>☐</td><td>☐</td><td>☐</td><td>☐</td><td>☐</td></tr>
<tr><td>Crowding in the incisor region</td><td>Spacing in the incisor region</td><td>Diastema in mm</td><td>Anterior maxillary misalignment in mm</td><td>Anterior mandibular misalignment in mm</td></tr>
</table>

***Alignment/Spacing No alignment-0 / 1-arch alignment-1 / 2-arch alignment-2**

<u>OCLUSION</u>

<table>
<tr><td>☐</td><td>☐</td><td>☐</td><td>☐</td></tr>
<tr><td>Over-emphasis in mm</td><td>Anterior crossbite in mm</td><td>Open bite anterior vertical in mm</td><td>**Anteroposterior molar relationship</td></tr>
</table>

****Normal molar ratio - 0 / Half cusp - 1 / Full cusp - 2**

$$\text{DAI} = (\text{Dentes perdidos} \times 6) + (\text{API}) + (\text{ESP}) + (\text{DI} \times 3) + (\text{DMXA}) + (\text{DMDA}) + (\text{OMXA} \times 4) + (\text{OMDA} \times 4) + (\text{MAA} \times 4) + (\text{RMAP} \times 3) + 13$$

Severity of malocclusion	Indication of treatment	DAI score
No abnormality or mild malocclusion	No or little need	≤25
Definite malocclusion	Elective	26 a 30
Severe malocclusion	Highly desirable	31 a 35
Very severe or disabling malocclusion	Indispensable	≥36

ANNEX F

Anteroposterior molar relationship:

- (O) normal;

- (1) mela cùspide (when the first molar was displaced mela cùspide - mesially or distally - in relation to its normal position);

- (2) whole cusp (when the first molar was displaced one cusp mesially or distally - in relation to the normal position).

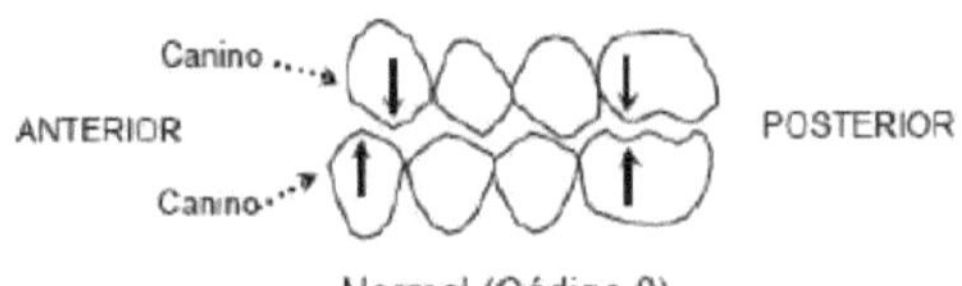

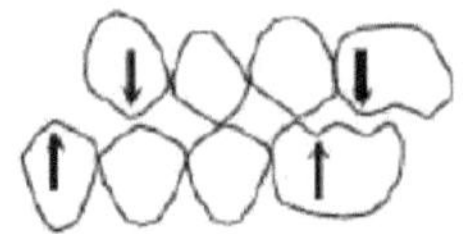

Molar inferior está a meia cúspide mesialmente de sua relação normal

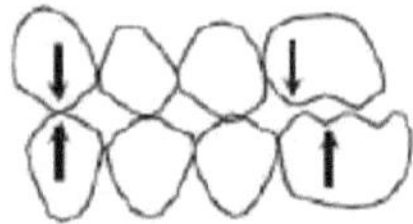

Molar inferior está a meia cúspide distalmente de sua relação normal

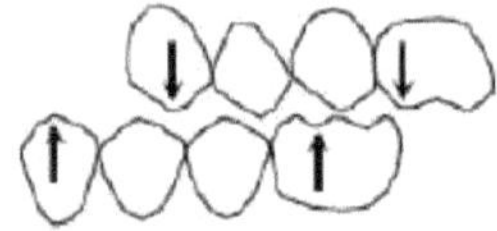

Molar inferior está a uma cúspide ou mais mesialmente de sua relação normal

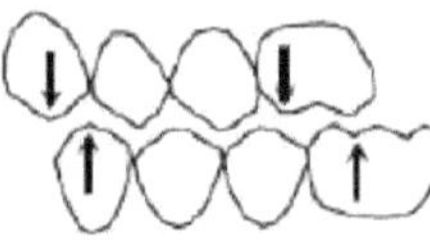

Molar inferior está a uma cúspide ou mais distalmente de sua relação normal

ANNEX G

QUESTIONNAIRE

Name:Date of birth ____ /____ / ____

Address: Phone:

Neighborhood: ____

City:

School you attend:Grade: Class:

Father's name:____

Mother's name: ____

QUESTIONS:

1 - Do you like your smile? ( ) 1.Yes ( ) 2. No ( ) 3.I don't know

2   - How do you feel about the appearance of your teeth?

( ) 1. Very satisfied - ( ) 2.Satisfied - ( ) 3.Unsatisfied -

( ) 4.Very dissatisfied - ( ) 5.Don't know

3   - How does your oral health affect your relationships with other people? ( ) I.It doesn't - ( ) 2.It affects a little - ( ) 3.It affects more or less -

( ) 4.Affects a lot -( ) 5.Don't know

4   - Is there anything you'd like to change about your teeth?

( ) 1.Yes - ( ) 2.No - ( ) 3.Don't know

5   - If yes, what would you like to change: ( ) 1.Color-- ( ) 2.Size - ( ) 3.Position - ( )4. Other:

( ) 4. nothing

6   - Do other people comment on the appearance of your teeth?

( ) 1.Yes, often - ( ) 2.Yes, sometimes - ( ) 3.No - ( ) 4.Don't know

7   - Do you avoid smiling because of the appearance of your teeth?

( ) 1. Yes, often - ( ) 2.Sometimes - ( ) - 3.Never - ( )4. I don't know

8   - Do you hide your mouth because of the appearance of your teeth?

( ) 1. yes, almost always - ( ) 2. yes, a few times - ( ) 3. never - ( ) 4. don't know

9   - Would you like to improve your smile?

( ) 1.Yes - ( ) 2.No - ( ) 3.Don't know

10   - Do you think you need orthodontic treatment?

( ) 1.Yes - ( ) 2.No - ( ) 3.Don't know

11   - Have you ever worn braces to fix the position of your teeth?

( ) 1.Yes, I've finished my treatment - ( ) 2.Yes, I'm in treatment -

( ) 3.No ( ) 4.Don't know

12   **- Visual analog scale** 0 10

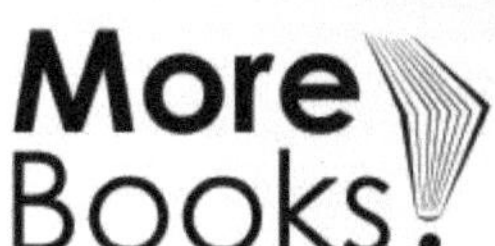

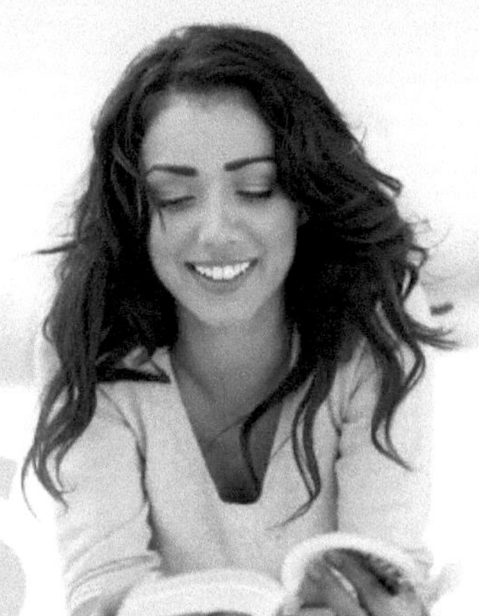

Buy your books fast and straightforward online - at one of world's fastest growing online book stores! Environmentally sound due to Print-on-Demand technologies.

Buy your books online at
www.morebooks.shop

Kaufen Sie Ihre Bücher schnell und unkompliziert online – auf einer der am schnellsten wachsenden Buchhandelsplattformen weltweit! Dank Print-On-Demand umwelt- und ressourcenschonend produziert.

Bücher schneller online kaufen
www.morebooks.shop

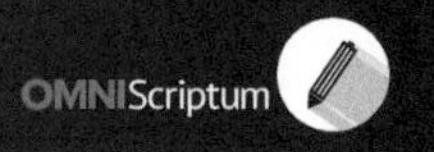

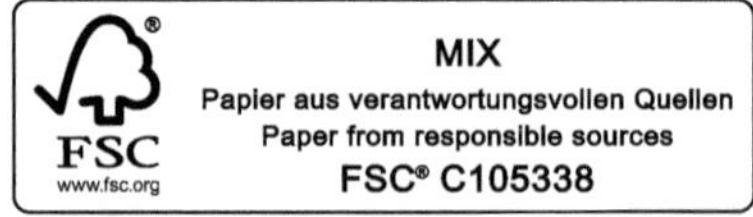

Printed by Books on Demand GmbH, Norderstedt / Germany